2024 STROKE DIET RECIPE COOKBOOK FOR BEGINNERS

Master Stroke Recovery: Recipes, Meal Plans, & Pantry Guide for a Healthy Future

Daniel J. Contreras

Table of Contents

Stroke and the Role of Diet in Recovery

When blood flow to the brain is interrupted, brain cells are deprived of oxygen and nutrients, which leads to a stroke.This can lead to cell death and damage, causing various symptoms depending on the affected brain region.

While there's no single "stroke recovery diet," dietary changes can play a crucial role in supporting healing and reducing the risk of future strokes. Here's how:

1. Promoting Cardiovascular Health:

- Fruits and Vegetables: Aim for at least five servings daily.

They are rich in antioxidants, vitamins, minerals, and fibre, which can help lower blood pressure, cholesterol, and inflammation, all contributing factors to stroke.

- Whole Grains: Opt for whole-grain bread, cereals, pasta, and rice over refined ones. Whole grains provide sustained energy, fibre for digestion, and essential nutrients.

- Lean Protein: Choose lean protein sources like fish, poultry, beans, and nuts. They are essential for building and repairing tissues, crucial for recovery.

- Healthy Fats: Include healthy fats like those found in olive oil, avocados, and nuts in moderation.

These fats are good for heart health and may even improve cognitive function.

2. Managing Specific Conditions:

- **High Blood Pressure:** Limit sodium intake by reducing processed foods, using herbs and spices for flavouring, and checking food labels for sodium content.
- **Diabetes:** Manage blood sugar levels through a balanced diet that includes complex carbohydrates, fruits, vegetables, and lean protein.

3. Addressing Swallowing Difficulties:

- **Food Texture: If swallowing is challenging, opt for softer foods like mashed potatoes, yoghurt, soups, and well-cooked vegetables.**
- **Hydration: Drink plenty of fluids throughout the day to prevent dehydration and aid swallowing.**

Additional Tips:

- **Portion Control: Focus on smaller, more frequent meals to ease digestion and improve nutrient absorption.**
- **Variety: Include a diverse range of foods from all food groups to ensure a balanced intake of essential nutrients.**

- **Seek Guidance:** Consult a registered dietitian or healthcare professional for personalised dietary advice tailored to your specific needs and medical conditions.

Getting Started with Your Stroke Recovery Journey: A Warm Welcome!

We understand that recovering from a stroke can be a challenging and overwhelming experience. But you're not alone! This cookbook is designed to be your companion on the road to a healthy future, offering delicious and nutritious recipes specifically tailored to support your stroke recovery journey.

Before we jump into the culinary delights, let's address some essential points:

- **Understanding your condition: This book will provide a brief overview of stroke and how diet plays a crucial role in your recovery. We'll explore the benefits of the DASH diet, which emphasises fruits, vegetables, whole grains, and lean protein, while limiting unhealthy fats, sodium, and added sugars.**
- **Essential nutrients: We'll delve into the importance of specific nutrients for stroke recovery, highlighting the benefits of incorporating fruits, vegetables, whole grains, and lean protein sources into your daily meals.**

- **Mind the salt:** Reducing sodium intake is crucial for post-stroke health. We'll offer practical strategies and tips to help you navigate this step.

- **Cooking techniques:** This section will equip you with essential cooking methods that are not only healthy but also create delicious and satisfying meals.

Part 1 Building a Strong Foundation for Recovery: The Power of Diet after Stroke

After experiencing a stroke, the road to recovery can seem daunting. But one powerful tool you have in your arsenal may surprise you: your diet!

Just like a strong foundation is crucial for building a sturdy house, a well-balanced diet plays a vital role in supporting your body's healing process after a stroke. This section of the book will guide you through the essential components of a stroke-friendly diet, explaining how each element contributes to your recovery.

First, let's explore the DASH Diet:

This acronym stands for Dietary Approaches to Stop Hypertension, and it's not just for people with high blood pressure! The DASH diet has been scientifically proven to be beneficial for overall cardiovascular health, which is crucial for stroke recovery. It emphasises:

- **Fruits and vegetables: Packed with vitamins, minerals, and antioxidants, these colourful gems play a vital role in fighting inflammation and promoting cell repair.**

- **Whole grains:** These complex carbohydrates provide sustained energy, helping you to stay active and engaged in your rehabilitation journey.
- **Lean protein:** Whether it's fish, poultry, or plant-based sources like beans and lentils, protein is essential for building and repairing tissues, vital for post-stroke recovery.

Now, let's address two key elements to limit in your diet:

- **Sodium:** Reducing your sodium intake is crucial for managing blood pressure, which lowers the risk of future strokes. We'll explore strategies for reducing hidden sodium in your meals.

- Unhealthy fats: Saturated and trans fats can contribute to inflammation and other health problems. We'll guide you towards choosing healthier fat sources like olive oil and avocado.

Building a Stroke-Friendly Plate:

Imagine your plate divided into three sections:

- Half filled with colourful fruits and vegetables.
- One quarter filled with whole grains or starchy vegetables.
- The remaining quarter is filled with lean protein.

This simple visual can help you create balanced and nutritious meals throughout your day.

Cooking Techniques for Success:

Healthy doesn't have to mean bland! We'll introduce you to cooking methods that are not only healthy but also enhance the flavor and enjoyment of your food. Think grilling, baking, steaming, and using herbs and spices for a taste explosion.

Chapter 1: Understanding the DASH Diet - Your Ally on the Road to Recovery

After experiencing a stroke, regaining your health and well-being becomes your top priority. While medication and rehabilitation play crucial roles, your diet can also be a powerful tool in your recovery journey. This chapter introduces you to the DASH diet, a scientifically proven approach that can benefit you significantly.

What is the DASH Diet?

DASH stands for Dietary Approaches to Stop Hypertension. Initially designed to manage high blood pressure, the DASH diet has been shown to offer much broader benefits, making it a valuable tool for post-stroke recovery.

How Does DASH Help Your Recovery?

The DASH diet emphasises:

- **Fruits and vegetables: Packed with vitamins, minerals, and antioxidants, these colourful gems play a vital role in reducing inflammation and promoting cell repair, both crucial for post-stroke healing.**

- **Low-fat dairy products:** These provide essential calcium, potassium, and protein, all contributing to bone health, blood pressure regulation, and muscle function.

- **Whole grains:** These complex carbohydrates offer sustained energy, aiding in physical and mental recovery.

- **Lean protein:** Whether from fish, poultry, or plant-based sources, protein is essential for rebuilding damaged tissues and supporting muscle strength, vital for regaining mobility and reducing the risk of future falls.

Benefits of DASH for Stroke Recovery:

- **Lowers blood pressure: One of the major risk factors for stroke is high blood pressure. By emphasising fruits, vegetables, and whole grains while limiting sodium, the DASH diet can help manage blood pressure, reducing the risk of future strokes.**

- **Improves cholesterol levels: The DASH diet encourages healthy fats while limiting saturated and trans fats, which can contribute to the buildup of plaque in your arteries. This can help improve your overall cardiovascular health and reduce the risk of future vascular problems.**

- **Supports weight management:
  Maintaining a healthy weight is crucial
  for reducing the risk of future strokes
  and overall cardiovascular health. The
  DASH diet promotes balanced eating
  and portion control, which can help
  you maintain a healthy weight.**

Making DASH Work for You:

This plan isn't a rigid set of rules, but a framework for healthy eating. You can customise it to fit your preferences and dietary needs. Remember, consistency is key. Start by incorporating small changes, such as adding more fruits and vegetables to your meals or opting for lean protein sources.

By understanding the principles of the DASH diet and incorporating its core components into your daily routine, you're taking a proactive step towards a healthier future, empowering your body to heal and regain strength after a stroke.

Chapter 2: Essential Nutrients for Stroke Recovery: Focus on Fruits, Vegetables, Whole Grains, and Lean Protein

After a stroke, your body needs the right fuel to rebuild and heal. This chapter delves into the essential nutrients that should be the stars of your stroke-friendly diet, focusing on the powerhouses: fruits, vegetables, whole grains, and lean protein.

Fruits and Vegetables: A Rainbow of Benefits:

Imagine a vibrant explosion of colours on your plate - that's the power of fruits and vegetables! These champions are packed with essential vitamins, minerals, and antioxidants.

- **Vitamins: Think A, C, and E, crucial for boosting your immune system and fighting inflammation, both key elements in stroke recovery.**
- **Minerals: Potassium, magnesium, and calcium play a vital role in regulating blood pressure, muscle function, and nerve transmission, all contributing to your overall well-being.**

- **Antioxidants: These superheroes fight free radicals, harmful molecules that can damage your cells. Including a variety of colourful fruits and vegetables in your diet ensures a good dose of these protectors.**

Whole Grains: The Powerhouse of Energy:

Ditch the refined carbs and embrace the world of whole grains! In contrast to refined grains, whole grains are loaded with:

- **Fibre: This keeps you feeling fuller for longer, aids in blood sugar control, and promotes gut health. All crucial factors for a healthy recovery journey.**

- **B vitamins:** These vitamins are essential for energy production, nervous system function, and maintaining a healthy metabolism.
- **Minerals:** Whole grains are a good source of magnesium, which helps regulate blood pressure and muscle function.

Lean Protein: Building Blocks for Repair:

Your body needs protein to rebuild damaged tissues and support muscle growth, both crucial for regaining strength and mobility after a stroke. Here are your lean protein options:

- Fish: Fatty fish like salmon, tuna, and sardines are excellent sources of omega-3 fatty acids, known for their anti-inflammatory properties and benefits for brain health.

- Poultry: Opt for skinless chicken or turkey breast for a lean protein source.

- Plant-based proteins: Beans, lentils, tofu, and tempeh are excellent plant-based alternatives, providing protein and fibre.

Putting it all Together:

Think of these essential nutrients as a team working together to support your recovery. By incorporating a variety of fruits, vegetables, whole grains, and lean protein into your daily meals, you're providing your body with the building blocks it needs to heal and thrive.

Tips for Success:

- Have a fruit and veggie smoothie to start your day.
- Pack colourful snacks like sliced bell peppers and carrots with hummus.
- Replace refined bread with whole-wheat options.
- Choose grilled or baked fish for a protein-rich dinner.

- **Try varying the herbs and spices you use to give your food more taste.**

Chapter 3: Mind Your Salt: Strategies for Reducing Sodium Intake in your Diet

Sodium, often referred to as salt, plays a crucial role in regulating bodily functions like blood pressure and fluid balance. However, excessive sodium intake is a major risk factor for high blood pressure, which can significantly increase the risk of stroke.

This chapter dives into the importance of reducing your sodium intake after a stroke and equips you with practical strategies to achieve this goal without compromising on flavour in your meals.

Why is Sodium Reduction Important After a Stroke?

Following a stroke, managing your blood pressure is crucial for preventing future complications. Consuming excessive sodium can cause your blood vessels to constrict, leading to higher blood pressure.

How Much Sodium Should You Aim For?

The American Heart Association recommends limiting your daily sodium intake to less than 2,300 milligrams (mg), ideally aiming for no more than 1,500 mg for optimal health, especially after a stroke.

Strategies to Reduce Sodium in Your Diet:

Become a Label Detective: Reading food labels is your first line of defence. Look for options labelled "low-sodium," "reduced-sodium," or "no salt added." Be mindful of serving sizes, as even low-sodium options can contain surprising amounts of sodium if you consume a larger portion.

Embrace Fresh and Frozen Options: Fresh fruits, vegetables, and unprocessed meats naturally contain little to no sodium. Opt for frozen options without added salt or sauce for convenience.

Cook More at Home: This gives you complete control over the sodium content of your meals. Explore herbs, spices, and other flavour enhancers like lemon juice, garlic, and vinegar to add depth and complexity without relying on salt.

Beware of Hidden Sodium Sources: Many seemingly healthy processed foods, like canned soups, condiments, and deli meats, can be loaded with sodium.

Be mindful when choosing these items and opt for low-sodium alternatives whenever possible.

Rinsing Canned Foods: Soaking or rinsing canned vegetables and beans can help remove some of the added sodium.

Gradual Reduction is Key: Don't try to go cold turkey! With time, gradually cut back on the amount of salt you use when cooking. Your taste buds will adjust, and you won't even miss the extra salt after a while.

Chapter 4: Cooking Techniques for Delicious and Stroke-Friendly Meals

Eating healthily doesn't have to be monotonous and tasteless.This chapter introduces you to a variety of cooking techniques that are not only healthy but also enhance the flavour and enjoyment of your stroke-friendly meals.

Embrace the Power of Heat:

- **Grilling and baking: These methods use minimal oil and allow the natural flavours of your food to shine through. Try grilling fish, chicken, or vegetables for a smoky and delicious twist.**

Baking is perfect for creating tender and flavorful casseroles, roasted vegetables, and lean protein sources.

- Sautéing and stir-frying: These techniques use a small amount of healthy oil to quickly cook your food while preserving its nutrients and texture. Perfect for creating stir-fries with colourful vegetables, lean protein, and whole grains.

Unlock the Magic of Liquids:

- Poaching and simmering: These gentle cooking methods use low heat and liquid to cook your food, resulting in juicy and tender results.

Poach fish, chicken, or tofu for a healthy and flavorful protein source. Simmer vegetables in broth or water to infuse them with delicious flavour.

- **Steaming: This healthy and versatile technique preserves the nutrients and vibrant colours of your vegetables. Steam broccoli, asparagus, or green beans for a quick and delicious side dish.**

Flavor Boosters Beyond Salt:

- **Herbs and spices: Explore the world of herbs and spices to add complexity and depth to your dishes without relying on salt. Experiment with rosemary, thyme, garlic powder, chili flakes, and countless other options to suit your taste preferences.**

- **Citrus: A squeeze of lemon or lime juice can brighten up your dishes and add a refreshing touch. Try marinating fish or chicken in citrus juice for added flavour.**

- **Acidity: A touch of vinegar or balsamic glaze can balance out sweetness and add a pleasant tang to your meals. Drizzle balsamic glaze over roasted vegetables or use a splash of vinegar in salad dressings.**

Additional Tips:

- **Invest in good quality cookware: This can make a world of difference in the outcome of your meals.**

A good non-stick pan can help you cook with minimal oil, and a versatile baking sheet can be used for endless healthy dishes.

- Utilise leftovers: Leftovers can be transformed into creative new meals. Leftover grilled chicken can be used in salads or wraps, and roasted vegetables can be added to omelettes or soups.
- Have fun and experiment! Try experimenting with different flavours and methods without fear.Cooking should be enjoyable, and with a little creativity, you can create delicious and healthy meals that support your stroke recovery journey.

Part 2: Recipes for Every Meal

Breakfast is often called the "most important meal of the day," and for good reason! It sets the tone for your metabolism and provides your body with the fuel it needs to kickstart your day. After a stroke, a nutritious breakfast is even more crucial for promoting recovery and supporting your overall well-being.

This chapter offers a variety of delicious and stroke-friendly breakfast recipes to suit your preferences and dietary needs:

1. Whole-wheat toast and spinach paired
with scrambled eggs:

This classic breakfast is packed with
protein, fibre, and essential vitamins.
Scramble two eggs with a splash of low-fat
milk. Sauté a handful of spinach with
minced garlic and add it to the eggs towards
the end of cooking. Season with pepper and
enjoy on a slice of whole-wheat toast.

2. Berry Smoothie Bowl:

Blend a cup of plain yoghurt with half a cup
of frozen berries and a splash of
unsweetened almond milk for a creamy and
refreshing base. Top with additional berries,
sliced banana, granola, and a sprinkle of
chia seeds for added texture and nutrients.

3. Whole-Wheat Pancakes with Greek Yogurt and Fruit:

Combine whole-wheat flour, baking powder, and a sprinkle of cinnamon in a bowl. Mix in a mashed banana, egg, and milk until well combined. Cook pancakes on a lightly greased pan. Top with a dollop of plain Greek yoghurt and your favourite sliced fruit like strawberries, blueberries, or mangoes.

4. Oatmeal with Nuts and Seeds:

Cook oats in water or low-fat milk according to package instructions. Top with chopped nuts like almonds or walnuts, a sprinkle of chia seeds, and a drizzle of honey for a touch of sweetness.

5. Cottage Cheese with Sliced Vegetables and Whole-Wheat Toast:

Spread a layer of low-fat cottage cheese on a slice of whole-wheat toast. Top with sliced cucumbers, tomatoes, and bell peppers for a light and refreshing start to your day.

Chapter 5: Breakfast: Jumpstart Your Day with Power-Packed Options

After a stroke, a nutritious breakfast takes on even greater significance. It sets the stage for your entire day, providing your body with the essential nutrients it needs to heal, rebuild, and regain strength. This chapter dives into a variety of delicious and stroke-friendly breakfast options to jumpstart your day with power!

Why is Breakfast Important After a Stroke?

- **Provides vital energy: After a night's rest, your body needs fuel to kick things off.**

A healthy breakfast helps stabilise blood sugar levels, providing sustained energy for your rehabilitation and daily activities.

- Supports brain health: Breakfast provides your brain with the nutrients it needs to function optimally, enhancing focus, memory, and cognitive function.

- Promotes muscle recovery: Protein-rich breakfasts help rebuild and repair muscle tissue, essential for regaining strength and mobility after a stroke.

Here are 5 delicious and nutritious breakfast recipes to kickstart your morning:

Recipe 1: Tropical Smoothie Bowl

Ingredients:

- 1 cup frozen mango chunks
- 1/2 cup frozen pineapple chunks
- 1/2 banana, frozen
- 1/2 cup plain Greek yoghourt
- 1/4 cup unsweetened almond milk
- 1 tablespoon chia seeds
- Toppings (optional): granola, sliced banana, fresh berries

Instructions:

1. Blend together the frozen mango, pineapple, banana, Greek yoghurt, and almond milk until smooth and creamy.

2. After transferring the smoothie into a bowl, add the toppings of your choice.

Nutritional Value (per serving):

-   Calories: 300
-   Protein: 15g
-   Carbs: 40g
-   Fat: 5g

Recipe 2: Scrambled Eggs with Spinach and Smoked Salmon

Ingredients:

- **2 eggs**
- **1 tablespoon milk**
- **1 handful of fresh spinach, chopped**
- **1 slice of smoked salmon, crumbled**
- **Salt and pepper to taste**
- **Olive oil spray**

Instructions:

1. **In a bowl, whisk the eggs and milk together..**
2. **Heat a pan with olive oil spray over medium heat.**

3. Cook the spinach for approximately a minute, or until it wilts.

4. Pour in the egg mixture and scramble with a spatula until cooked through.

5. Top with crumbled smoked salmon, salt, and pepper.

Nutritional Value (per serving):

- **Calories: 250**
- **Protein: 20g**
- **Carbs: 2g**
- **Fat: 15g**

Recipe 3: Overnight Oats with Berries and Nuts

Ingredients:

- 1/2 cup rolled oats
- 1/2 cup milk (dairy or non-dairy)
- 1/4 cup plain Greek yoghourt
- 1/4 cup berries (fresh or frozen)
- 1 tablespoon chopped nuts (almonds, walnuts, etc.)
- 1 teaspoon honey (optional)

Instructions:

1. In a jar or container, combine the rolled oats, milk, Greek yoghurt, berries, nuts, and honey (if using).
2. Stir well, cover, and refrigerate overnight.
3. Enjoy the cold in the morning.

Nutritional Value (per serving):

- Calories: 300
- Protein: 10g
- Carbs: 40g
- Fat: 10g

Recipe 4: Whole-Wheat Toast with Avocado and Eggs

Ingredients:

- 1 slice whole-wheat bread
- 1/2 avocado, sliced
- 2 eggs
- Salt and pepper to taste
- Olive oil spray

Instructions:

1. Toast the whole-wheat bread.
2. Mash the avocado and spread it on the toast.
3. Heat a pan with olive oil spray over medium heat.
4. Fry the eggs to your desired doneness.
5. Place the eggs on top of the avocado toast and season with salt and pepper.

Nutritional Value (per serving):

- **Calories: 350**
- **Protein: 15g**
- **Carbs: 30g**
- **Fat: 15g**

Recipe 5: Breakfast Burrito with Sweet Potato and Black Beans

Ingredients:

- 1 whole-wheat tortilla
- 1/2 cup roasted sweet potato cubes
- 1/4 cup black beans, rinsed and drained
- 1 scrambled egg
- 1 tablespoon salsa
- 1/4 cup chopped avocado (optional)

Instructions:

1. The whole-wheat tortilla can be warmed in a microwave or pan..

2. Spread the salsa on the tortilla.

3. Top with the roasted sweet potato cubes, black beans, scrambled egg, and avocado (if using).

4. Enjoy the tortilla after folding it into a burrito.

Nutritional Value (per serving):

- Calories: 350
- Protein: 15g
- Carbs: 40g
- Fat: 10g

Chapter 6: Lunch: Light and Nutritious Meals for Midday

As the day progresses, maintaining your energy levels is crucial for continued rehabilitation and recovery after a stroke. Lunch plays a vital role, offering an opportunity to refuel with light, nutritious meals that won't weigh you down or leave you feeling sluggish. This chapter explores a variety of delicious and stroke-friendly lunch options to keep you energised and empowered throughout your afternoon.

Why is a Healthy Lunch Important After a Stroke?

- **Sustains energy levels: Balanced meals help maintain stable blood sugar levels, preventing energy crashes that can hinder your recovery and daily activities.**

- **Supports muscle recovery: Protein-rich lunches provide essential building blocks for muscle repair and strength restoration, crucial for regaining mobility and reducing the risk of falls.**

- **Boosts cognitive function: Choosing foods rich in essential vitamins and minerals can enhance focus, memory, and cognitive function, aiding in your overall well-being.**

Fuel your afternoon with these delicious and satisfying lunch options, each packed with essential nutrients to keep you energised and focused.

1. Mediterranean Chickpea Salad Pita Pockets (Vegetarian, Gluten-free adaptable):

- Ingredients:
    1. 1 can (15 oz) of rinsed and drained chickpeas
    2. 1/2 cucumber, diced
    3. 1/2 red bell pepper, diced
    4. 1/4 red onion, diced
    5. 1/4 cup crumbled feta cheese (omit for vegan)
    6. 2 tablespoons chopped fresh parsley
    7. 2 tablespoons olive oil
    8. 1 tablespoon lemon juice

9. 1/2 teaspoon dried oregano

10. Salt and pepper to taste

11. 2 whole wheat pitas (corn tortillas for gluten-free)

- Nutritional Value (per serving): Calories: 350, Fat: 13g, Carbohydrates: 35g, Protein: 15g

- Instructions:

    1. In a bowl, combine chickpeas, cucumber, bell pepper, onion, feta cheese (if using), and parsley.

    2. Whisk together olive oil, lemon juice, oregano, salt, and pepper in a separate bowl.

    3. Drizzle the salad with the dressing and toss to coat.

    4. Warm the pitas (or tortillas) and fill with the chickpea salad.

2. Spicy Salmon Sushi Bowls:

Ingredients:

1. 4 oz cooked salmon, flaked
2. 1 cup cooked brown rice
3. 1/2 avocado, sliced
4. 1/4 cup shredded carrots
5. 1 tablespoon crumbled seaweed (optional)
6. 1 tablespoon sriracha mayo (or mix 1 tbsp sriracha with 1 tbsp mayonnaise)
7. 1 tablespoon soy sauce
8. 1 teaspoon sesame oil
9. As a garnish, add chopped green onions and sesame seeds (optional).

Nutritional Value (per serving): Calories: 450, Fat: 20g, Carbohydrates: 40g, Protein: 30g

Instructions:

10. In a bowl, combine brown rice, salmon, avocado, carrots, and seaweed (if using).
11. In a small bowl, whisk together sriracha mayo, soy sauce, and sesame oil.
12. Drizzle the sauce over the bowl and toss to coat.
13. Optionally garnish with green onions and sesame seeds.

3. Lentil Soup with Whole Wheat Toast:

- **Ingredients:**

  - 1 tablespoon olive oil
  - 1 medium onion, chopped
  - 2 cloves garlic, minced
  - 1 carrot, chopped
  - 1 celery stalk, chopped
  - 1 cup brown lentils, rinsed
  - 4 cups vegetable broth
  - 1 (14.5 oz) can diced tomatoes, undrained
  - 1 teaspoon dried thyme
  - 1/2 teaspoon dried oregano
  - Salt and pepper to taste
  - 2 slices whole wheat bread, toasted

- **Nutritional Value (per serving): Calories: 300, Fat: 8g, Carbohydrates: 45g, Protein: 15g**

Instructions:

- In a big pot, warm up the olive oil over medium heat.
- . Add onion, garlic, carrot, and celery and cook until softened, about 5 minutes.
- Add lentils, broth, tomatoes, thyme, oregano, salt, and pepper. Once the lentils are cooked, simmer for 20 to 25 minutes on low heat after bringing to a boil.

4 . Serve hot with toasted whole wheat
bread.

4. Greek Quinoa Salad with Chicken:

- Ingredients:

    1. 1 cup cooked quinoa
    2. 1 grilled chicken breast, chopped
    3. 1/2 cup crumbled feta cheese
    4. 1/4 cup cherry tomatoes, halved
    5. 1/4 cup kalamata olives, sliced
    6. 1/4 red onion, thinly sliced
    7. 1 cucumber, diced
    8. 1 tablespoon chopped fresh parsley
    9. 2 tablespoons olive oil
    10. 1 tablespoon lemon juice

11. 1/2 teaspoon dried oregano

12. Salt and pepper to taste

- **Nutritional Value (per serving): Calories: 400, Fat: 15g, Carbohydrates: 30g, Protein: 35g**

- **Instructions:**

1. In a large bowl, combine quinoa, chicken, feta cheese, tomatoes, olives, onion, cucumber, and parsley.

Chapter 7: Dinner: Delicious and Satisfying Dishes for the Whole Family

The end of the day is a time to connect with loved ones and unwind. This chapter focuses on creating delicious and satisfying dinner options that are not only stroke-friendly but also cater to the whole family.

Sharing meals with family and friends can:

- Boost enjoyment: Eating together can make healthy meals more enjoyable, especially when you share the experience with loved ones.

- **Promote healthy habits:** By incorporating healthy meals into your family routine, you encourage healthy habits for everyone, not just yourself.

- **Create lasting memories:** Sharing meals can foster connection, conversation, and create lasting memories for everyone involved.

Delicious and Stroke-Friendly Dinner Ideas:

- **Salmon with Roasted Vegetables:** Baked salmon is a fantastic source of lean protein and omega-3 fatty acids, beneficial for heart and brain health. Roast a variety of colourful vegetables like broccoli, carrots, and bell peppers for a vibrant and nutrient-rich side dish.

- Turkey Chili with Brown Rice: This hearty chili is packed with protein from ground turkey, fibre from kidney beans, and vitamins from vegetables like tomatoes, corn, and onions. Serve it with brown rice for added fibre and complex carbohydrates.

- Chicken Stir-Fry with Whole-Wheat Noodles: Stir-frying is a quick and healthy cooking method that allows you to retain the nutrients in your vegetables. Combine lean chicken with colourful vegetables like broccoli, snap peas, and red peppers. Serve it over whole-wheat noodles for a satisfying and balanced meal.

- **Lentil Shepherd's Pie:** This vegetarian option is just as flavorful and comforting as the classic. Lentils provide protein and fibre, while mashed potatoes offer a creamy and satisfying topping. Add chopped vegetables like carrots, peas, and corn for additional flavour and nutrients.

- **Baked Cod with Lemon Herb Sauce:** Cod is a mild-flavoured white fish that's perfect for baking. Drizzle it with a light lemon herb sauce for a flavorful and healthy meal. Pair it with roasted vegetables or quinoa for a complete and balanced dinner.

Tips for Creating Family-Friendly Meals:

- **Involve the whole family: Get your family involved in meal planning, preparation, and even setting the table. This creates ownership and promotes healthy habits for everyone.**

- **Offer choices: Provide a variety of healthy options within each food group to cater to individual preferences and dietary needs.**

- **Focus on flavour: Make healthy meals taste delicious! Experiment with herbs, spices, and different cooking methods to create exciting flavours your family will enjoy.**

- **Make it fun: Set the table with colourful plates and napkins, play some music, and enjoy the company of your loved ones.**

Here are 5 delicious and light lunch recipes to keep you energised throughout the afternoon:

Recipe 1: Mediterranean Tuna Salad Sandwich

Ingredients:

1 can (5 oz) of drained tuna in water

1 can (5 oz) tuna in water, drained

1/4 cup chopped cucumber

1/4 cup chopped tomato

1/4 cup crumbled feta cheese

1 tablespoon olive oil

1 tablespoon lemon juice

Salt and pepper to taste

Instructions:

1. In a bowl, combine tuna, cucumber, tomato, feta cheese, olive oil, lemon juice, salt, and pepper.

2. Spread the mixture on one slice of bread and top with the other slice.

Nutritional Value (per serving):

- Calories: 350
- Protein: 20g
- Carbs: 30g
- Fat: 15g

Recipe 2: Lentil Soup with Whole-Wheat Croutons

Ingredients:

- 1 tablespoon olive oil
- 1 onion, chopped
- 2 cloves garlic, minced
- 1 carrot, chopped
- 1 celery stalk, chopped

- 1 cup brown lentils, rinsed

- 4 cups vegetable broth

- 1 can (14.5 oz) diced tomatoes, undrained

- 1 teaspoon dried oregano

- Salt and pepper to taste

- 2 slices whole-wheat bread, cubed and toasted

Instructions:

1. In a pot, warm the olive oil over medium heat.. Add onion, garlic, carrot, and celery, and cook until softened, about 5 minutes.

2. Stir in lentils, vegetable broth, diced tomatoes, and oregano. Once the lentils are cooked, simmer for 20 to 25 minutes on low heat after bringing to a boil.

3. Season with salt and pepper to taste.

4. Serve soup with whole-wheat croutons on top.

Nutritional Value (per serving):

- **Calories: 300**
- **Protein: 15g**
- **Carbs: 40g**
- **Fat: 10g**

Recipe 3: Chicken Salad with Grapes and Walnuts

Ingredients:

- **2 cups cooked shredded chicken**
- **1/2 cup green grapes, halved**
- **1/4 cup chopped walnuts**
- **1/4 cup mayonnaise (light or Greek yoghourt)**

- 1 tablespoon Dijon mustard

- 1 tablespoon lemon juice

- Salt and pepper to taste

- Lettuce leaves (optional)

Instructions:

1. In a bowl, combine shredded chicken, grapes, walnuts, mayonnaise, Dijon mustard, lemon juice, salt, and pepper.

2. Serve on lettuce leaves or in a whole-wheat wrap.

Nutritional Value (per serving):

- Calories: 400

- Protein: 30g

- Carbs: 20g

- Fat: 20g

Recipe 4: Rainbow Veggie Wrap with Hummus

Ingredients:

- 1 whole-wheat tortilla
- 1/4 cup hummus
- 1/4 cup shredded carrots
- 1/4 cup chopped cucumber
- 1/4 cup chopped bell peppers
- 1/4 cup baby spinach
- Salt and pepper to taste

Instructions:

1. Spread hummus on the whole-wheat tortilla.
2. Layer carrots, cucumber, bell peppers, and spinach on top.
3. Season with salt and pepper to taste.
4. Roll up the tortilla tightly and enjoy.

Nutritional Value (per serving):

- Calories: 300
- Protein: 10g
- Carbs: 40g
- Fat: 10g

Recipe 5: Edamame Salad with Brown Rice and Sesame Ginger Dressing

Ingredients:

- 1 cup cooked brown rice

- 1 cup shelled edamame, cooked and cooled
- 1/2 cup chopped cucumber
- 1/4 cup chopped red onion
- 1 tablespoon sesame oil
- 1 tablespoon rice vinegar
- 1 teaspoon soy sauce
- 1 teaspoon grated ginger
- Salt and pepper to taste

Instructions:

1. In a bowl, combine brown rice, edamame, cucumber, and red onion.
2. In a separate bowl, whisk together sesame oil, rice vinegar, soy sauce, ginger, salt, and pepper.
3. Drizzle the salad with the dressing and toss to coat..

Nutritional Value (per serving):

- Calories: 350
- Protein: 15g
- Carbs: 45g
- Fat:

Chapter 8: Snacks: Healthy Nibbles to Keep You Going Throughout the Day

After a stroke, maintaining consistent energy levels is crucial for supporting your recovery and overall well-being. While three balanced meals are essential, healthy snacks can play a vital role in keeping you fueled and energised throughout the day.

This chapter dives into a variety of delicious and stroke-friendly options to keep your body and mind nourished between meals.

Why are Healthy Snacks Important After a Stroke?

- **Prevent energy dips: Small, healthy snacks throughout the day help stabilise blood sugar levels, preventing sudden drops that can lead to fatigue and hinder your recovery efforts.**

- Provide essential nutrients: Snacks can bridge the gap between meals, ensuring your body receives a constant supply of essential vitamins, minerals, and protein for continued healing and repair.

- Support muscle recovery: Opting for protein-rich snacks can help maintain muscle mass and support muscle recovery, crucial for regaining strength and mobility.

Tips for Smart Snacking:

- **Plan ahead: Preparing healthy snacks in advance prevents reaching for unhealthy options when hunger strikes.**

- **Portion control: Avoid overdoing it. Stick to planned portion sizes to prevent consuming excess calories.**

- **Pay attention to your body and only eat when you're genuinely hungry—not when you're bored or responding to feelings.**

- Choose wisely: Opt for snacks that offer a combination of protein, fibre, and healthy fats.

- Hydrate: Don't mistake thirst for hunger. Water consumption throughout the day can help reduce mindless munching.

By incorporating these healthy and delicious snack options into your routine, you can ensure your body receives the consistent fuel it needs to support your recovery journey and maintain energy levels throughout the day.

Here are 5 delicious and healthy snack recipes to keep you fueled throughout the day:

Recipe 1: Trail Mix with a Twist

Ingredients:

- 1/2 cup raw almonds
- 1/4 cup dried cranberries
- 1/4 cup dark chocolate chips
- 1/4 cup pumpkin seeds
- 1 tablespoon shredded coconut (optional)

Instructions:

1. In a bowl, combine almonds, cranberries, chocolate chips, pumpkin seeds, and coconut (if using).
2. Mix well and store in an airtight container.

Nutritional Value (per serving):

- **Calories: 250**
- **Protein: 5g**
- **Carbs: 20g**
- **Fat: 15g**

Recipe 2: Roasted Chickpeas with Herbs and Spices

Ingredients:

- 1 can (15 oz) chickpeas, drained and rinsed
- 1 tablespoon olive oil
- 1/2 teaspoon dried oregano
- 1/4 teaspoon chili powder
- 1/4 teaspoon garlic powder
- Salt and pepper to taste

Instructions:

1. Preheat the oven to 400°F (200°C).
2. Pat chickpeas dry with a paper towel.
3. In a bowl, toss chickpeas with olive oil, oregano, chili powder, garlic powder, salt, and pepper.
4. Spread chickpeas on a baking sheet in a single layer.

5. Roast for 20-25 minutes, or until golden brown and crispy.

6. Let cool slightly before serving.

Nutritional Value (per serving):

- Calories: 200
- Protein: 8g
- Carbs: 20g
- Fat: 5g

Recipe 3: Greek Yoghourts Parfait with Berries and Granola

Ingredients:

- 1 cup plain Greek yoghourt
- 1/4 cup mixed berries (fresh or frozen)
- 2 tablespoons granola

Instructions:

1. Layer Greek yoghurt, berries, and granola in a small bowl or parfait glass.
2. Repeat layers if desired.
3. Enjoy immediately.

Nutritional Value (per serving):

- Calories: 250
- Protein: 15g
- Carbs: 30g
- Fat: 5g

Recipe 4: Edamame with a Spicy Kick

Ingredients:

- 1 cup shelled edamame, frozen or fresh
- 1 teaspoon olive oil
- 1/4 teaspoon chili flakes
- Pinch of salt

Instructions:

1. If using frozen edamame, cook according to package directions.
2. Heat olive oil in a pan over medium heat.
3. Add edamame and chili flakes and cook for 2-3 minutes, stirring occasionally.

4. Sprinkle it with salt and serve immediately.

Nutritional Value (per serving):

- Calories: 150

- Protein: 10g

- Carbs: 10g

- Fat: 5g

Recipe 5: Apple Slices with Almond Butter

Ingredients:

- 1 apple, sliced

- 2 tablespoons almond butter

Instructions:

1. Slice the apple.

2. Spread almond butter on the apple slices.

3. Enjoy!

Nutritional Value (per serving):

- **Calories: 200**
- **Protein: 5g**
- **Carbs: 25g**
- **Fat: 10g**

Part 3: Planning and Maintaining a Stroke-Friendly Lifestyle

Building a Brighter Future: Planning and Maintaining a Stroke-Friendly Lifestyle

Regaining your health and well-being after a stroke is an ongoing journey. While medication and rehabilitation play crucial roles, adopting a stroke-friendly lifestyle is equally important in ensuring your long-term health and preventing future complications. This section equips you with the tools and resources to plan and maintain a lifestyle that empowers your recovery and promotes overall well-being.

Chapter 9: Sample Meal Plans for Different Dietary Needs:

This chapter provides sample meal plans tailored to different dietary needs, including:

- Low-sodium options: This plan offers strategies to maintain a healthy diet while managing sodium intake.
- Vegetarian and vegan options: Discover delicious and nutritious plant-based meals that are both stroke-friendly and satisfying.

- **Diabetic-friendly options:** Learn how to incorporate healthy and balanced meals into your routine while managing diabetes, a risk factor for stroke.

Chapter 10: Building a Stroke-Friendly Pantry: Essential Ingredients to Keep on Hand:

This chapter serves as your guide to stocking your pantry with essential ingredients that are versatile and can be easily incorporated into stroke-friendly meals. These include:

- **Whole grains: Brown rice, quinoa, whole-wheat pasta, and oats offer complex carbohydrates and fibre for sustained energy.**
- **Lean protein sources: Skinless chicken and turkey breast, fish (especially fatty fish like salmon),**

beans, lentils, and tofu are essential
for muscle repair and recovery.

- Fruits and vegetables: Stock up on a
variety of colourful fruits and
vegetables to ensure a constant intake
of essential vitamins, minerals, and
antioxidants.

Healthy fats: Olive oil, avocado, and
nuts provide healthy fats essential for
heart health and cognitive function.

- Low-sodium options: Look for
low-sodium broths, canned
vegetables, and condiments to manage
your sodium intake.

Chapter 11: Tips for Managing Grocery Shopping and Meal Preparation:

This chapter guides you through planning your grocery shopping and meal preparation to ensure you have healthy and delicious options readily available:

- Plan your meals: Create a weekly menu to avoid impulse purchases at the grocery store.

- Make a grocery list: Stick to your list and avoid getting sidetracked by tempting but unhealthy options.

- **Prepare meals in advance:** Batch cooking or preparing ingredients in advance saves time and ensures you have healthy options readily available.

- **Read food labels:** Pay close attention to portion sizes and sodium content when choosing packaged foods.

- **Don't be afraid to experiment:** Explore new recipes and cooking techniques to keep your meals exciting and enjoyable.

Conclusion

Embracing a Healthy Lifestyle: Your Key to Stroke Prevention

The effects of a stroke can be life-altering, making prevention a crucial aspect of maintaining long-term health. While some risk factors are beyond our control, many can be mitigated by adopting a healthy lifestyle. This guide empowers you to take charge of your well-being and significantly reduce your risk of stroke.

Key Pillars of a Stroke-Preventive Lifestyle:

1. Maintain a Healthy Weight: Being overweight or obese is a major risk factor for stroke.

    Use a balanced diet and frequent exercise to help you reach your ideal weight.

    2 .Eat a Balanced Diet: Embrace a diet rich in fruits, vegetables, and whole grains. Limit unhealthy fats, processed foods, added sugars, and excessive salt intake. Opt for lean protein sources and healthy fats from nuts, seeds, and olive oil.

2. Engage in Regular Exercise: Try to get in at least 150 minutes a week of moderate-to-intense aerobic activity or 75 minutes a week of strenuous

activity.Even small increases in physical activity can significantly benefit your health.

3.Manage Stress: Chronic stress can contribute to high blood pressure, a major risk factor for stroke. Practice stress-management techniques like yoga, meditation, or deep breathing exercises to keep stress levels in check.

4. Limit Alcohol Consumption: Excessive alcohol intake can raise blood pressure and increase your stroke risk. Moderate alcohol

consumption is generally defined as one drink per day for women and two drinks per day for men.

However, it's important to consult your doctor about the right amount for you, and even complete abstinence may be recommended in some cases.

5. Quit Smoking: Smoking is one of the most significant risk factors for stroke. Quitting smoking significantly reduces your risk and improves your overall health. Please don't hesitate to ask for help; there are lots of resources available to assist you with quitting.

6.Manage Existing Medical Conditions: If you have high blood pressure, high cholesterol, diabetes, or atrial fibrillation, work closely with your doctor to manage these conditions effectively. By controlling these conditions, you significantly reduce your risk of stroke.

7. Regular Checkups: Schedule regular checkups with your doctor to monitor your blood pressure, cholesterol levels, and blood sugar. Early detection and treatment of any underlying health conditions can significantly reduce your stroke risk.